Summer Drinks

2nd Edition

16 Quick & Easy Drink Recipes That Will Cool You Down in The Summer

by Olivia Rogers

Copyright © 2017 By Olivia Rogers
All rights reserved. No part of this book may be reproduced in any form without permission in writing from the author. No part of this publication may be reproduced or transmitted in any form or by any means, mechanic, electronic, photocopying, recording, by any storage or retrieval system, or transmitted by email without the permission in writing from the author and publisher.
For information regarding permissions write to author at Olivia@TheMenuAtHome.com
Reviewers may quote brief passages in review.

Please note that credit for the images used in this book go to the respective owners. You can view this at:
ArtsCraftsAndMore.com/image-list

Olivia Rogers
TheMenuAtHome.com

Table of Contents

Introduction _____ *4*

1. Sunrise Margarita _____ *5*

2. June Bug _____ *8*

3. Cucumber Sangria _____ *10*

4. Blackberry Lemonade _____ *12*

5. Peach Punch _____ *15*

6. Watermelon Daiquiri _____ *19*

7. Pisco Sour _____ *21*

8. Lemonade _____ *23*

9. Minty Iced Tea _____ *25*

10. Rose Collins _____ *27*

11. Tropical Smoothie _____ *29*

12. Coconut and Strawberry Cream Soda _____ *31*

13. Carrot Lemonade _____ *33*

14. Melon Heat Quenchers _____ *35*

15. Watermelon Punch _____ *37*

16. Raspberry Lemonade _____ *39*

Final Words _____ *41*

Disclaimer _____ *43*

Introduction

Summer is a time that everyone looks forward to. They are excited for the warm days that seem to last so much longer than normal, yet not long enough.

The time that they get to hang out with family and friends and do the things that they love, or at least get chores done outside around the house.

But when you are done with all of that hard work or hard play, it is time to sit back and relax before hydrating that body.

Instead of just drinking plain water or running out of ideas on what to serve at your next party, check out these delicious recipes in this guidebook.

Give a few a try and enjoy the tastes that summer has to offer.

1. Sunrise Margarita

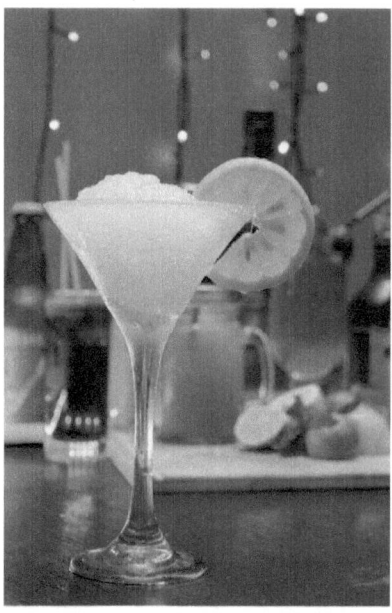

This is such an easy and great to look at cocktail that will give you all of the flavors to remind you of summer, no matter what time of year it is.

Add some red sugar to the rim of your cup to get a great fiery look that is all its own.

Ingredients

- Red sugar

- 1 wedge of lime

- 2 c. orange liqueur

- 1 ½ c. lime juice

- 2 c. tequila

- 2 c. orange juice

- 1 c. powdered sugar

- Grenadine syrup

- Orange slices

- Ice cubes

Method

1. To start this recipe, place some sugar onto a plate and have it all spread out. Rub the rims of your glasses with a lime wedge before dipping into the sugar and getting all coated. Set to the side.

2. Bring out a big pitcher and combine the sugar, lime juice, tequila, and triple Sec. Stir so that the sugar dissolves and then stir the orange juice. Chill in the fridge until you are ready to serve.

3. Place the ice cubes into your prepared glasses before pouring in the juice mixture and adding 2 sprits of the grenadine syrup. Garnish with the slices of orange if you would like before serving.

Notes

The flavors that come in the glass can give you a bright colorful look that is fun for the beach or just relaxing on your porch. Many people find that it is nice for their BBQ's as well. If you need a non-alcoholic beverage, you can remove the tequila and still get a great taste.

2. June Bug

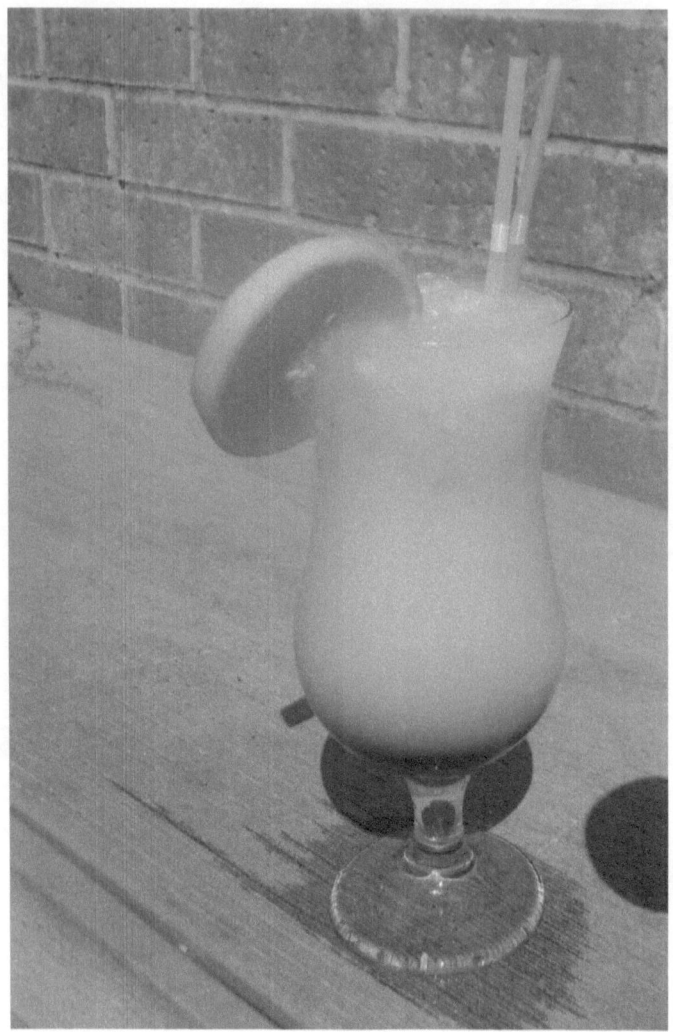

Not every drink for the summer needs to be filled with alcohol and this is a great example. It has some bubblies and some sugar sweetness to fill any hearts' desire and can be enjoyed by kids and adults alike.

Ingredients

- 4 Tbsp. grenadine
- 3 c. ginger ale
- 3 scoops orange sherbet
- 4 Tbsp. orange juice

Method

1. To begin this recipe, blend the sherbet, orange juice, grenadine together until they are nice and smooth.
2. Pour this into some cocktail glasses that have some ice in them and then enjoy.

Notes

If you are serving this at a kids' party or just to your children in the summer, leave the recipe as it is. On the other hand, you can also make this drink more adult friendly by adding in a little bit of white rum.

3. Cucumber Sangria

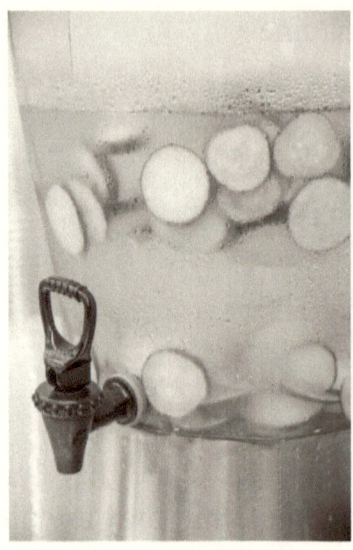

Nothing can cool you down on a hot summers' day than some fresh cucumbers. This drink is a great way to get them in, so you can stay refreshed while still getting in your healthy vegetable nutrition. What could be better than that?

Ingredients

- 1 sliced seedless cucumber
- 1 honeydew melon
- 1 sliced lime
- ¼ c. lime juice
- 12 mint leaves, fresh

- ¼ c. honey

- 1-liter chilled carbonated water

- 1 bottle dry white wine

Method

1. To begin this recipe, cut the melon up so that it is in half. Remove and then get rid of the rind and the seeds so that you just have the fruit left. Cut up the rest of the melon so that you have slices. Bring out the pitcher that you have and combine the mint leaves, lime slices, cucumber, and melon inside and set to the side.

2. Take out a bowl and stir together both the honey and the lime juice until they are well combined. Pour over the mixture in the pitcher before adding the wine and stirring a bit. Cover the pitcher and let this drink chill for a minimum of 2 hours. When you are ready to serve, add in the carbonated water of your choice. Ladle this into glasses and then serve.

Tips

This mixture is going to make quite a bit of the drink. If you find that you do not have enough room in your fridge for the whole drink, split it up into smaller containers to use some now and some later.

4. Blackberry Lemonade

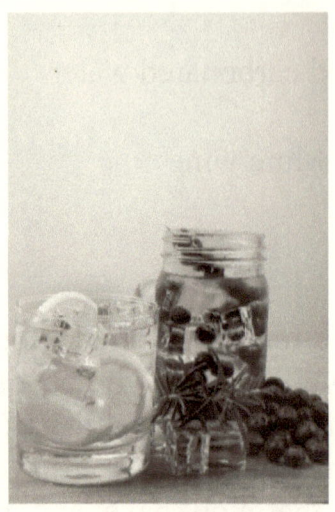

Fruity drinks are the favorites in summer. They taste so good and can add so much refreshment that it can be really difficult to put them down. This one is especially popular, and you can make it either with or without the alcohol for your needs.

Ingredients

- 1 ½ Tbsp. lemon juice

- ¼ c. bourbon

- 1/3 c. chilled sparkling lemonade

- 13 oz. blackberries

- ¾ c. water

- ¼ c. sugar

- 1 ½ Tbsp. rosemary

Method

1. The first thing that you should work on is the syrup for the drink. To do this, take out a saucepan and combine the sugar, water, rosemary, and blackberries. Bring this to a boil before reducing the heat and letting this simmer for about 25 minutes.

2. After this time, you can mash up the blackberries and then take the pan from the heat. Allow to cool down before straining through a strainer and into a jar that has been cleaned. Try to get as much liquid out as possible. You can use it to make the drink right away or store for a week.

3. When you are ready to make the drink, bring out a cocktail shaker. Combine the ice, a few tablespoons of the syrup you made, lemon juice, and bourbon. Shake this for around 30 seconds in order to mix and chill the ingredients. Strain this into some glasses that are filled with ice. Top the mixture with some sparkling lemonade and then garnish with a few blackberries if you would like.

Tips

If you want to save some time you can combine the lemonade, lemon juice, and bourbon into a glass with some ice and then pour the syrup in to get the colors how you would like.

It is also possible to make a big batch of this drink if you would like to have it for a party. To do this add in a whole recipe of the syrup with 2/3 cups of the lemon juice, and 3 cups bourbon. Add in 4 cups of the lemonade and garnish with the blackberries. This will make 12 servings.

5. Peach Punch

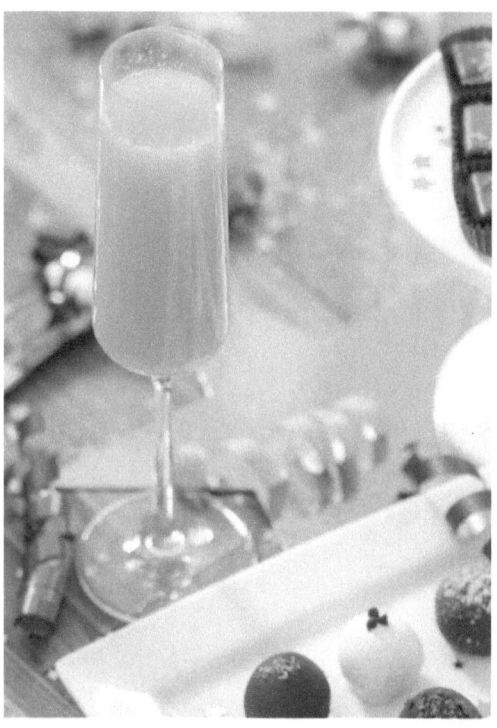

Summer is the time to meet up with friends and family and you never know when someone is going to stop by. This peachy mixture is perfect for throwing into the freezer and pulling out whenever someone shows up unexpectedly.

Ingredients

- 1 ½ c. sugar

- 3 c. water

- 1 can peaches in syrup, sliced

- 1 pkg. gelatin, peach flavored

- ½ c. lemon juice

- 4 cans peach nectar

- 8 bottles ginger ale

Method

1. Take out a pan and combine the gelatin, sugar, and water. Stir and bring to a boil until the sugar and the gelatin until they are dissolved. Next you can bring out a blender and place the peaches inside. Cover the blender and blend these until they become smooth.

2. Now you need a really big bowl and combine the lemon juice, peach nectar, pureed peaches, and gelatin mixture together. Divide up the peach mixture between 4 containers which are a quart each. Cover and let this freeze until it is firm. You can leave in there for 3 months if you would like to have it ready whenever anyone comes.

3. When you are ready to serve, take one of the containers out of the freezer and let it set at a room temperature for an hour. After this time, break it into chunks using a fork and then place inside a jug or a punch bowl. Stir in 2 of the ginger ale bottles for each of the containers you use and then mix so it becomes a slushy. Serve right away.

Tip

This is a recipe that is pretty big because it is meant for a storage to use over time. If you would like to use a smaller amount, just halve or quarter the recipe and then make the mixture after freezing just for the night. You can also make the mixture bigger if needed for a large party.

Read This FIRST - 100% FREE BONUS

FOR A LIMITED TIME ONLY – Get Olivia's best-selling book *"The #1 Cookbook: Over 170+ of the Most Popular Recipes Across 7 Different Cuisines!"* absolutely FREE!

Readers have absolutely loved this book because of the wide variety of recipes. It is highly recommended you check these recipes out and see what you can add to your home menu!

Once again, as a big thank-you for downloading this book, I'd like to offer it to you *100% FREE for a LIMITED TIME ONLY!*

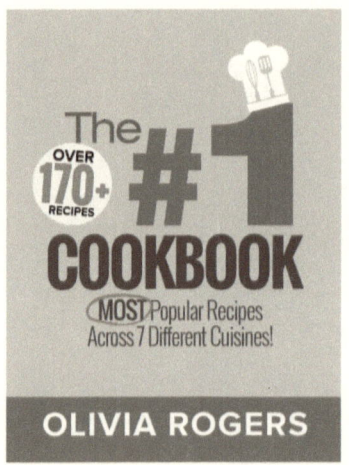

Get your free copy at:

TheMenuAtHome.com/Bonus

6. Watermelon Daiquiri

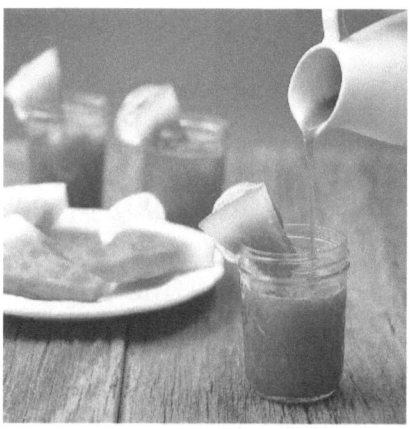

Nothing says summer better than a little bit of watermelon and this drink is going to have you wishing that the beautiful weather never goes away. Shake up the summer a bit with this naturally sweet juice that has a bit of crispness added with the punch of flavor that comes with the basil and rum add to it. Take a taste and see how great summer can be.

Ingredients

- 6 cubes of watermelon

- ¼ c. light rum

- 4 basil leaves

- 1 ½ Tbsp. syrup

- 2 Tbsp. lime juice

- ¼ c. water

- ¼ c. sugar

Method

1. To begin this recipe, you will need to make the syrup. TO do this you should bring out a pan and combine the water and the sugar. Bring this to a light boil, stirring the whole time in order to let the sugar dissolve. Cool this down and let chill for an hour before you use it.

2. Once the syrup is done, take out a cocktail shaker. Combine together the basil and the watermelon and muddle so the watermelon becomes juiced.

3. At this time, add in the ice, simple syrup you made, lime juice, and rum. Shake some more to get it chilled, which will take around 40 seconds. Double strain this into some glasses filled with ice. Garnish with a little extra watermelon and then serve this drink right away.

Tips

It is easy to make this into a bigger batch if you would need to serve a larger group. Just make sure to double or triple the ingredients to get the amount that you want. Everyone at the party is going to enjoy the refreshing taste of the drink and you will be the talk of the party.

7. Pisco Sour

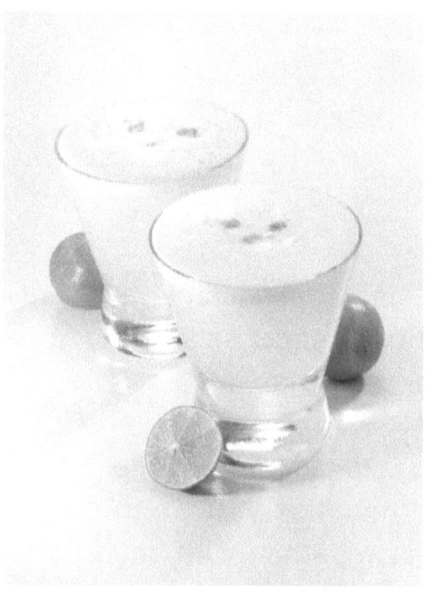

This is a fun cocktail that is going to give you a flavor that is so intense and so fresh that you will not be prepared for it thanks to the mixture of the lime and the mint. It is possible to make it an alcoholic drink with the pisco or to replace that with some sparkling water for those who just want something refreshing without the alcohol.

Ingredients

- 1 c. guava nectar

- 1 c. white rum or pisco (replace with sparkling water if going nonalcoholic).

- 2 tsp. superfine sugar

- Lime wedges

- Mint leaves

- Angostura bitters

Method

1. To start this simple recipe, take out a glass pitcher. Place the lime juice, sugar, guava nectar, and either the rum or the pisco.

2. Now you can add in a little bit of the Angostura bitters, as much as you would like and then stir the ingredients together well in order to let the sugar dissolve.

3. When ready to serve, divide up this mixture between 4 glasses of your choice. Add in the ice before topping with the mint and the lime wedge.

Tips

Place this drink into the fridge and let it cool down for a couple of hours before serving. This is better than using ice cubes because it allows the drink to be chilled without getting watered down from the ice.

8. Lemonade

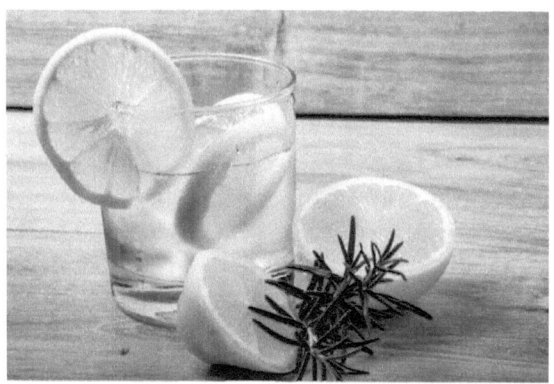

A classic favorite that everyone can remember from when they were kids. Whether you grew up in the deep south or went to visit your grandmother in the country of the Midwest, there is always sure to be some great tasting lemonade available upon request. And now that you are all grown up, it is possible to try this new peach variety to get some of the old tastes that you enjoyed as a child with a new twist.

Ingredients

- ¾ c. sugar
- 1 c. lemon juice
- 3 c. cold water
- Lemon slices
- Ice cubes

Method

1. To begin this recipe, you can bring out a pitcher and add the sugar, lemon juice, and water. Stir this until the sugar has been completely dissolved

2. If you would like, place into the fridge to chill a bit. Serve over some ice and garnish with a few slices of lemon.

Tips

The recipe listed above is for the traditional lemonade that you grew up loving. A new way to produce this tasty drink is to add in some peachy flavor. To do this place half of a can of peach slices into the blender with a cup of your lemonade. Blend to get it smooth before pouring into the pitcher. Repeat with the rest of the peaches and then serve with some ice cubes.

9. Minty Iced Tea

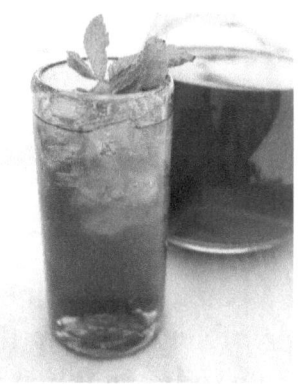

Tea just breathes the taste of summer and you will be able to get so many health benefits and great tastes when you use tea as the base ingredients. The next time that you are entertaining for the summer and need something cool and refreshing that everyone will enjoy, pull out this great recipe and be the hit of the party.

Ingredients

- 2 c. sugar
- 7 c. water
- 8 orange pekoe tea bags
- 8 c. water, cold
- 8 mint sprigs
- 2 c. orange juice

- Ice cubes

- Mint sprigs for garnish

- ¾ lemon juice

Method

1. First, take out a pan and combine the 7 cups of water with the 2 cups of sugar. Bring this to a boil and stir in the sugar to dissolve and then reduce the heat. Let this simmer for 5 minutes.

2. After this time, you can take it from the heat and add in the 8 sprigs of mint and the tea bags. Cover the pan and allow it stand for about 5 minutes. After this time remove the sprigs of mint and the tea bags with a spoon and discard them.

3. Transfer the heat to a big container before adding in the lemon juice, orange juice, and the remaining cold water. Cover the bowl and let it set in the fridge for a minimum of 4 hours. When you are ready to serve, place some ice in a few cups, pour the tea, and then garnish with mint sprigs if you would like.

Tips

This is a very large recipe of tea. If you are just serving for a smaller group and do not need as much tea, it is easy to halve the recipe to get the amount that you need.

10. Rose Collins

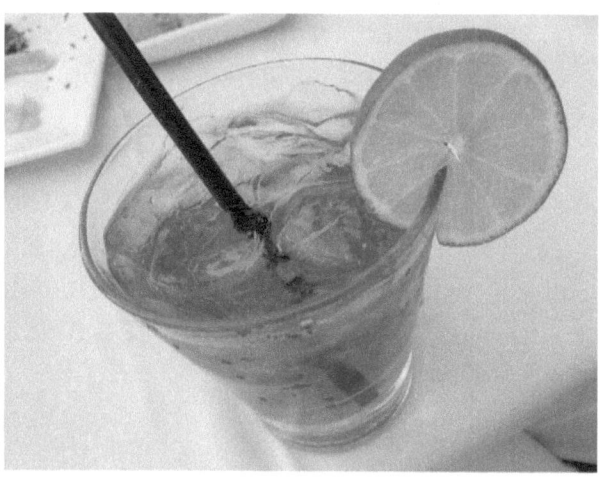

The first thing that you will notice about this drink is the floral smells and flavors that come with it. If it is a bit too girly for you, add a bit of Campari tames bitters in order to tame it all down to your preference.

Ingredients

- 3 Tbsp. vodka

- 2 Tbsp. rose syrup

- Lemon wheel, thin

- 1 tsp. Campari

- Chilled club soda and seltzer water

- Coarse sugar

Method

1. To start this recipe, bring out a cocktail shaker and combine the ice, Campari, rose syrup, and vodka. Shake for 30 seconds so that it is chilled.

2. When this is done, double strain it before placing into a Collins glass that is filled with ice. Top with the seltzer. Right before you serve, float the lemon wheel into it and then sprinkle on the coarse sugar over it all.

Tips

If you are looking for a drink that is a little more sour and tart for your enjoyment, you can add in a bit of homemade sour mix. To make this sour mix, you can combine a simple syrup with lime juice and lemon juice in equal parts. Combine this in the cocktail shaker with the rest of the ingredients and then serve with this extra kick.

11. Tropical Smoothie

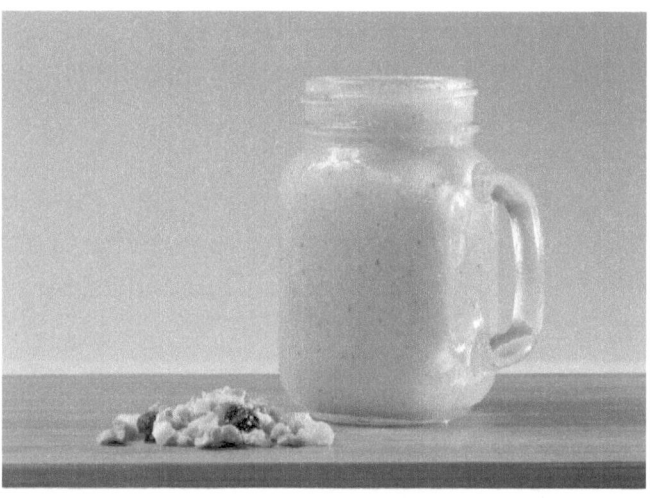

Take a vacation back to the islands this summer, even if you are stuck in the middle of the country. This is a great drink to enjoy either in the summer or in the winter and can give you a nice vacation away from it all.

Ingredients

- ½ c. chilled pineapple juice
- ½ frozen peeled bananas
- ½ c. chopped mango
- 1 Tbsp. lime juice
- ½ c. ice cubes

Method

1. For this recipe, you will need to bring out the blender. Place the lime juice, pineapple juice, banana, and mango inside.

2. Cover the blender and let it all blend so it becomes smooth. Slowly add in the ice and then continue to blend so you get the right consistency before serving.

Tips

You get to choose how creamy or smooth you would like the drink to be. If you like to have it with more of a juice like consistency, add in a few more ice cubes and blend for a bit longer. On the other hand, if you are interested in getting a smoother and creamier drink, add in a little bit more of the banana.

12. Coconut and Strawberry Cream Soda

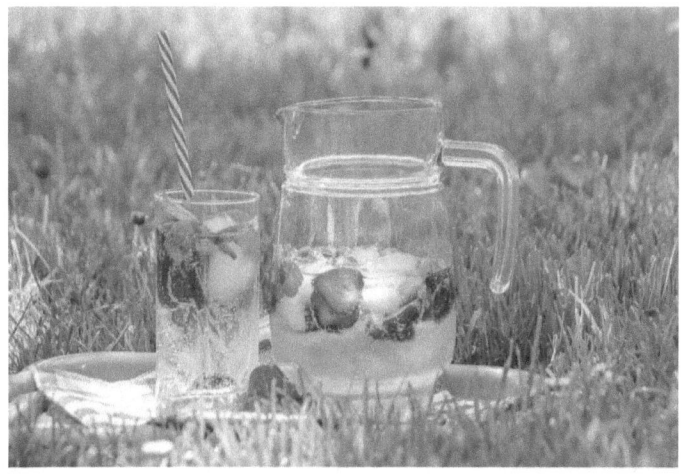

Coconut drinks are great because they can cool you down and get you all refreshed and ready to face the summer heat. You should look for some of the coconut milks in the grocery store to use for some of these delicious drinks.

Ingredients

- 2/3 c. sugar
- 3 c. halved strawberries
- 3 c. chilled carbonated water or club soda
- ¾ c. coconut milk, refrigerated.

Method

1. To begin this recipe, bring out a bowl and combine the sugar and the strawberries. Stir them well in

order to cover the strawberries. Once you are done with this, bring out a pastry blender and mash the strawberries coarsely.

2. Place about 1/3 cup of the berries into the bottom of six glasses. Add in some ice, a bit of club soda, and some coconut milk into each of the glasses. Right before you are ready to serve, you can stir the drinks and then enjoy.

Tips

This is a great drink to have at a summer gathering or to cool off after working hard around the house or the garden. Double this recipe so that you have some stored up when needed. It is best to only store for a few days or you can freeze to get it to last a bit longer.

13. Carrot Lemonade

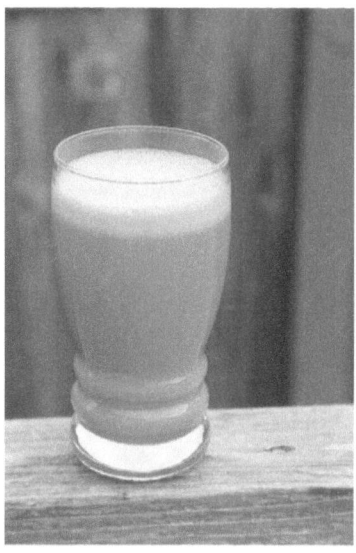

While the name might sound like it is a little bit out there, this lemonade is the one that you will need to make plenty of because the whole family will be asking for more. The best part is all of the healthy vitamins and minerals found inside that can keep your family strong and healthy for a long time to come.

Ingredients

- 2 c. water

- 1 lb. peeled and cut carrots

- ¾ c. lemon juice

- 3 c. pineapple juice

- Ice

- Cold water

- Lemon wedges

Method

Bring out a pan and combine the water and the carrots. Bring this to a boil before reducing the heat and covering it. Simmer these ingredients for about 30 minutes so the carrots can become tender.

When this is done, cool the mixture a bit before moving over to a blender. Add in a cup of the pineapple juice, cover the blender, and blend the ingredients until smooth. Once the ingredients are the consistency that you would like, transfer to a plastic container allow to chill in the fridge for a few hours before serving.

Tips

This is a great way to sneak in some extra vegetables to your children's meals. This can be tricky but when the carrots are hidden, they will be begging for more. Look for sugar free pineapple juice in order to get some extra benefits out of the process.

14. Melon Heat Quenchers

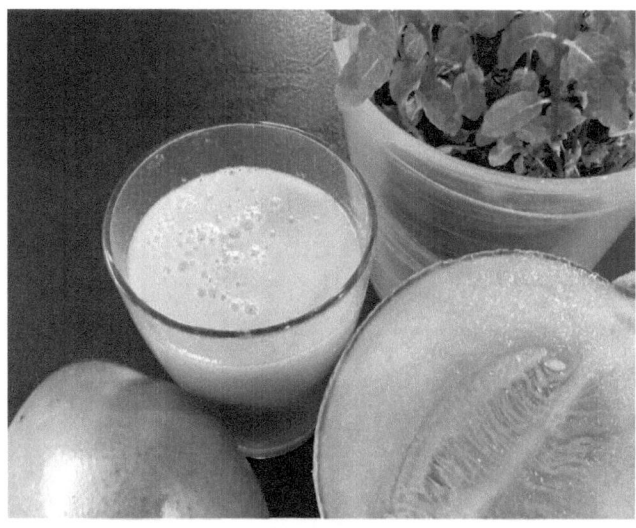

Melons come in so many different tastes and varieties that you are sure to find that one that will suit your mood. Check out this recipe and replace any melon that you want for something very unique.

Ingredients

- 3 ice cubes
- 1 c. watermelon, honeydew, or cantaloupe puree
- Plain yogurt
- ¼ grated ginger slice
- 1 tsp. honey

- Sparkling water (can have flavored if prefer)

- Lime peel, shredded

Method

1. To begin, puree the melon of your choice. To do this, chop up the melon and then place into a blender. Cover the blender and then turn on the machine to blend until fruit becomes smooth. You may need to stop a few times to push the mixture down and get it completely smooth.

2. Once that is done, add in the honey, a few teaspoons of yogurt, ginger, and ice cubes. Blend just to get the mixture smooth and frothy. Pour this into a serving glass and add some more honey if you would like. Stir the lime peel next to taste and then fill up the rest of the glass with the sparkling water.

Tips

If you would like to add a little treat or snack to the drink you can make some melon skewers. To do this, you can scoop out the melon of your choice into little balls. Thread them onto the wooden skewers before laying on a baking sheet and freezing for a few hours. Serve with the drink.

15. Watermelon Punch

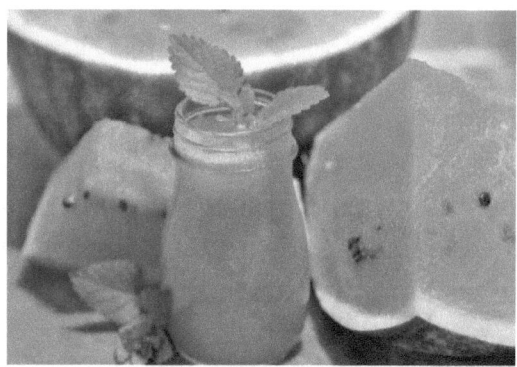

A tasty punch can spell the success of any summer day. Mixing a bit of watermelon with club soda, mint, sugar, lime juice, and white grape juice will give you the most festive drink you can find this summer in no time.

Ingredients

- ¾ c. watermelon

- 3 c. chopped and seeded watermelon

- ½ c. mint leaves, fresh

- 1 tsp. lime peel, shredded

- 2 c. white grape juice

- 32 oz. chilled club soda

- ¾ c. chilled lime juice

- Watermelon balls

- Mint sprigs

Method

1. To star this recipe, place the watermelon into a blender. Cover and let it blend for a few minutes so it becomes smooth. Strain this puree through a sieve and get rid of the pulp. Take out a bowl and combine together the mint and the sugar. Use a wooden spoon to crush the mint and press it to the side of your bowl.

2. At this time, add in the watermelon puree, lime juice, lime peel, and grape juice. Stir these ingredients until the sugar has dissolved. Add in the club soda. Pour this into glasses with some ice and garnish with the watermelon balls and mint sprigs before enjoying.

Tips

For a fun fruity taste, add in some more fruits to the juice. Strawberries and grapes are a great option, but you can also use other types of melon for more flavor.

16. Raspberry Lemonade

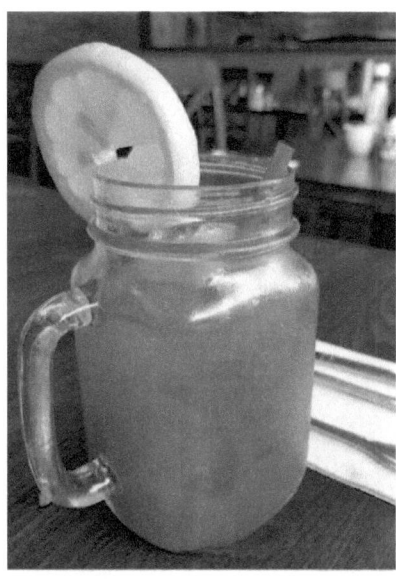

Nothing is as refreshing as a nice glass of lemonade when the summer heat gets to you, especially when you add in the light and fruity taste of raspberries. Keep a pitcher of this juice handy to enjoy whenever you get a hankering for the taste of summer.

Ingredients

- 12 oz. lemonade concentrate
- 18 oz. club soda
- 12 oz. vodka, pinnacle raspberry
- 1/8 c. grenadine

- Raspberries for garnish

- Lemon wedge, for garnish

Method

1. For this recipe, take out a pitcher and combine the regular ingredients together well. Put the pitcher into the fridge and let it chill for a few hours before serving.

2. When you are ready to serve this juice, pour it into a few glasses that have ice in them and then enjoy.

Tips

When you do not have a measuring glass available, use the can for the lemonade concentrate to help with measuring. You will need one full can for the vodka amount and one and a half cans for the club soda amount.

Final Words

I would like to thank you for downloading my book and I hope I have been able to help you and educate you about something new.

If you have enjoyed this book and would like to share your positive thoughts, could you please take 30 seconds of your time to go back and give me a review on my Amazon book page!

I greatly appreciate seeing these reviews because it helps me share my hard work!

Again, thank you and I wish you all the best with your cooking journey!

Last Chance to Get YOUR Bonus!

FOR A LIMITED TIME ONLY – Get Olivia's best-selling book *"The #1 Cookbook: Over 170+ of the Most Popular Recipes Across 7 Different Cuisines!"* absolutely FREE!

Readers have absolutely loved this book because of the wide variety of recipes. It is highly recommended you check these recipes out and see what you can add to your home menu!

Once again, as a big thank-you for downloading this book, I'd like to offer it to you *100% FREE for a LIMITED TIME ONLY!*

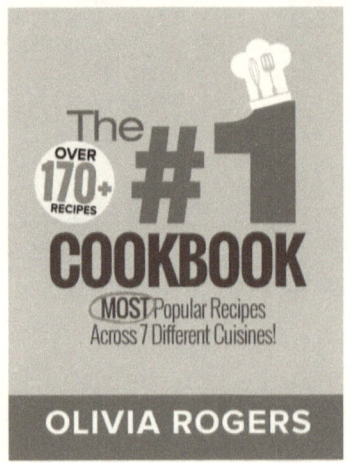

Get your free copy at:

TheMenuAtHome.com/Bonus

Disclaimer

This book and related site provides recipe and food advice in an informative and educational manner only, with information that is general in nature and that is not specific to you, the reader. The contents of this book and related site are intended to assist you and other readers in your personal efforts. Consult your physician or nutritionist regarding the applicability of any information provided in our information to you.

Nothing in this book should be construed as personal advice or diagnosis, and must not be used in this manner. The information provided about conditions is general in nature. This information does not cover all possible uses, actions, precautions, side-effects, or interactions of medicines, or medical procedures. The information in this site should not be considered as complete and does not cover all diseases, ailments, physical conditions, or their treatment.

No Warranties: The authors and publishers don't guarantee or warrant the quality, accuracy, completeness, timeliness, appropriateness or suitability of the information in this book, or of any product or services referenced by this site.

The information in this site is provided on an "as is" basis and the authors and publishers make no representations or warranties of any kind with respect to this information. This site may contain inaccuracies, typographical errors, or other errors.

Liability Disclaimer: The publishers, authors, and other parties involved in the creation, production, provision of information, or delivery of this site specifically disclaim any responsibility, and shall not be held liable for any damages, claims, injuries, losses, liabilities, costs, or obligations including any direct, indirect, special, incidental, or consequences damages (collectively known as "Damages") whatsoever and howsoever caused, arising out of, or in connection with the use or misuse of the site and the information contained within it, whether such Damages arise in contract, tort, negligence, equity, statute law, or by way of other legal theory.

www.ingramcontent.com/pod-product-compliance
Lightning Source LLC
Chambersburg PA
CBHW021134080526
4587CB00012B/1284